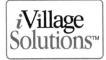

Best Advice on

LIFE AFTER BABY ARRIVES

Sleep, Sex, Sanity—and More!

Real Moms Share Practical Tips
That Worked for Them

Foreword by NANCY EVANS

RUTLEDGE HILL PRESS™

Nashville, Tennessee

A DIVISION OF THOMAS NELSON, INC.

www.ThomasNelson.com

Published by Rutledge Hill Press, a division of Thomas Nelson, Inc.,
P.O. Box 141000, Nashville, Tennessee 37214.

Library of Congress Cataloging-in-Publication Data is available

ISBN 1-4016-0043-3

Printed in the United States of America

03 04 05 06 07 — 5 4 3 2 1

CONTENTS

~

FOREWORD

By Nancy Evans

When I was pregnant with my daughter, a woman who was known for being a great mother sat me down to give me some of her good advice. One of the things she told me was that while everyone talks about what you should do for the baby, very few people think about what you should do for the mother.

So she gave me tips, like wearing a girdle after you give birth to help make your stomach flat again. (Can't say I did that, and the results show I didn't. But I'll pass it along to you.) She said to get a "mommy nurse." Meaning: *someone to take care of you, the new, exhausted mom. The baby needs care, but so do you.* This was news to me, and news that made huge sense. A beleaguered mom is not a happy mom; in fact, she's a mom who could get resentful and depressed. My "mommy nurse" was my mother; yours could be your best friend, great-aunt, or sister. The point is, don't try to go it alone.

I'll tell you something else. My favorite baby present was the box that came with stuffed animals for my daughter and nestled in tissue at the bottom of the box were silk pajamas for ME! And what those silk pajamas signaled to me was that I was still a woman, maybe even one who still had the potential for a sex life. I've made it a point ever since to always give a personal present to the new mom when I give a present to the baby.

That's what this book is about: It's the mother-care book to go along with all those baby-care books that we have piled up on the bedside table. This is the book that tells you how to take care of *you*. How to define yourself and continue to be a woman, a wife, a friend. No small thing. And, happily, there are plenty of women who have come through those first trying months of motherhood and have all sorts of good advice on how to remember that you're still a big part of the equation.

So sit back and make this book as much a part of your baby reading as the usual baby-care books. You—and everyone else in your life— will be the happier for it.

PREFACE

Since iVillage was founded in 1995, thousands of women have come to the discussion groups on the Website and asked other moms for help on life after the baby arrives. They've sought answers on keeping their sanity, getting some sleep, losing the baby weight, even how to ease back into sex. In this book, you'll find the very best solutions women have shared with one another in iVillage's online play groups, new mothers' circles, and support groups. The advice in this book is straight from the women of iVillage and provided by them as very real answers to the very real problems other moms have gone through.

iVillage would like to thank the members of its parenting communities for sharing their words of wisdom and inspiration. Without them, this book would not exist. We'd also like to thank the hundreds of community leaders who host our online discussion and support groups for the care, concern, and support they provide to our visitors and members. Danielle Brantley, Mary Curtis, Tawny Fadial, Robin Falck, Kathy Ohling, Joellyn Santo Paulo, Wendy Sybert, Corrine Sandusky, Susan Taylor, and Mitzi Trout provided invaluable assistance in helping us gather advice from the members of the iVillage community. And finally, many thanks to Kate Hanley for translating those many strains of online conversation into this book.

CHAPTER 1

How to Take Care of Yourself

"*I* ended up having panic attacks right after I had my first baby, because I didn't see a light at the end of the tunnel. Well, here I am with four kids, and I can tell you it does get better. What you're going through now isn't what things will always be like. Don't let anyone, especially you, make you feel guilty for doing something for yourself."

GET THE REST YOU NEED

"I am so tired. I feel like I never get the things done that I'd like to. Am I just feeling sorry for myself or are we all this tired?" —K.M.

"When I had my first baby, I thought I was the only one who felt insane from exhaustion. You may be surprised to know that almost everyone in this motherhood boat is as tired and worn out as you are. All parents start to question their sanity, especially that week before their kids start to sleep through the night. Give yourself a break. It's all the norm."

"Remember that just because your baby is awake, you don't have to coo over him every minute of the day."

"*I* used to get extremely tired until I decided that at least three nights during the week, I would go to bed when my daughter went to bed—between 7:30 and 8:00 P.M. It has made a big difference and gives me more energy on the other nights to stay up later and relax or get stuff done. I still get really tired, but I am better off than when I tried to stay up and do everything."

"My obstetrician of 25 years has a saying I love: 'Don't stand when you can sit. Don't sit when you can lie down. Don't stay awake if you can be asleep.' Take care of yourself at least half as well as you are taking care of your baby, and you will make it through."

"Be sure that when the baby naps, you nap. Even if you can't fall asleep, lie down and rest."

DON'T FEEL GUILTY ABOUT SCHEDULING "ME TIME"

"My problem with taking 'me time' is that I usually feel guilty thinking about the kids and how my husband is doing with them while I'm gone. How do I get over the guilt about having 'me time'? I can think of several things I would like to do, but the guilt is so strong." —M.S.

"To get over the guilt, start by taking five minutes every day to do something that's just for you—even if it's only sitting and doing nothing. Then add another five minutes, and keep adding. Eventually, you'll realize that everyone is surviving just fine without you and the guilt will go away."

"If you can't bring yourself to take scheduled time away from the baby, use her nap time as your 'me time.' Set up a box with things you like to do—cross-stitching, scrapbooking, crossword puzzles, whatever—and keep it nearby so you have it on hand when that free time arises. When the baby gets up, put your stuff in the box, and you're good to go."

"*G*et up 30 minutes earlier than everyone else and make it clear to everyone in the house that this is your time."

"*G*et your husband to take the kids out and away from you for a change. My husband did that and left 'strict instructions' that I was not to do any housework or anything for the rest of them because that time was for me."

"*I* keep my daughter in day care part-time, so I can have 'me time' each week. Sometimes I just run errands. Other times I meet a friend for lunch, go to an afternoon movie, or just lounge on the couch. I feel so rejuvenated after those days and so happy to see my daughter when I pick her up. Arrange for some help — if part-time child care doesn't work for you, then swap baby-sitting with another mom, so you can have some time off."

ACCEPT THAT YOU'VE DONE YOUR BEST (AND THAT'S ENOUGH)

"I have so much that I need to do, I just end up feeling overwhelmed. Any ideas or advice would be greatly appreciated!" —L.R.

"If you can answer the following questions with a yes, then relax already! Is your baby gaining weight? Is your pediatrician pleased with the way your baby is growing? Is your baby mostly content? Then don't worry."

"Remember, you just had a baby, and your whole life just changed. Give yourself some time to adjust to it all, and you will see in good time what is important."

"The curse of parenting is that you never feel like you're doing enough. Every day after I put my son to bed I think I could have read more to him, talked on the phone less, played more in the sandbox. It's hard to feel satisfied at the end of the day that you've done everything you could. You have to give yourself permission not to be the perfect parent, because such a thing just doesn't exist."

"*D*on't try to be perfect. Just try to organize a little, laugh a lot, and reach out for help if you need it."

"*T*aking care of babies and making them feel safe is the hardest job. You can feel truly incompetent until you look down at that tiny sleeping face and realize that you are the only one who can do the job. That's how important you are."

CHAPTER 2

How to Love the Shape You're In (While Getting Your Old One Back)

"The day my third child was born I weighed in at 181 pounds. I'm five-foot-three-inches! Almost two years later, I'm around 122 to 123 pounds. I've lost my weight by eating healthy and working out with videos at home (early in the morning before the kids get up) and running in the evenings."

$\mathcal{B}$E PROUD OF YOUR BODY—
THE WAY IT IS

*"How long until my body goes back to its
pre-pregnancy shape? I have so many weird fat
spots: My rings still don't fit, and my belly is not
what it used to be. When will I start to feel and
look normal again instead of like a recently
pregnant woman?"* —T.M.

"It's such a shame that we women feel so awful about our bodies. The women in magazines and movies aren't a very good representation of the wide variety of body types. I've had saggy breasts and stretch marks since I was 14. So now that I am the 31-year-old mother of a beautiful toddler, I finally feel like it's okay to have this body."

"The ideal figure in our society would be just like my lean, muscular, long-limbed seven-year-old's, but with boobs. That's ridiculous! Enjoy your kids, and relax with the rest of us. As long as you're physically and emotionally healthy, you're better off than just being thin."

"Sure I miss my pre-baby body, but there's no use in crying over it. That extra tummy skin and a few stretch marks are here to stay. But I have learned to appreciate the extra pounds and the lack of perfection. It has made me much more sympathetic toward people with less-than-outstanding bodies and less envious of women with terrific figures. I look back and wonder why I had nothing better to think about."

"It was really not that long ago that having a heavy wife was considered a sign of wealth and status. Just be healthy, that's what is really important. Besides, stretch marks are not scars—they are badges of courage. You've earned them."

"Before having my daughter, I was always worried about losing weight. Since her birth I have become accepting of my body and all its bumps, bruises, and lumps. Giving birth was, in many ways, a very empowering experience for me. As soon as I stopped worrying about my weight, I dropped down to my pre-pregnancy weight. My waist is thicker, but that isn't an issue. My confidence has improved 100 percent."

$\mathcal{A}$CCEPT THAT YOU'LL LOSE WEIGHT AT YOUR OWN PACE

"My scale has not moved since my baby was born. I walk four miles, five days a week. I eat very healthy food, and I am nursing exclusively. My best friend had her baby the same week as me, and she is back to her pre-pregnancy weight. She has not worked out once and eats everything she wants. How can it be so different for people?" —J.M.

"*I*'ve had three babies and it always takes me a year to lose the last six pounds. The good news is that after a year it comes off and then some. Eating healthfully and exercising get everything into shape nicely. It is hard not to become frustrated, but keep doing what you are doing and ignore the scale; it will pay off in the end."

"*I* have decided not to worry about weight loss while I'm nursing my daughter. Try to be happy being in shape and eating as best you can and be glad with small triumphs—I zipped up a coat recently and that made my day!"

"*I* really hate the pressure society puts on us to get rid of all the weight as though it is something shameful and we need to erase all signs of being pregnant as quickly as possible. It takes nine months to put it on, and it's going to take at least that to take it off. As long as you are exercising and eating healthy, good for you!"

"*My* experiences with weight loss were vastly different with each of my two children. With my daughter, I didn't lose a pound until she was weaned, and then the weight seemed to just melt off. With my son, I've not only managed to lose all my pregnancy weight within a few months, but I'm 12 pounds below my pre-pregnancy weight."

"Don't wait too long, like I did. I kept nursing and everyone would say, 'Oh, wait until he's three months old, you'll really start losing,' or, 'Wait until he's six months old, it will kick in.' I have finally started a diet and have lost about five pounds. If you're several months postpartum and you haven't lost anything yet, find a reputable diet that works for you."

CREATE NEW EXERCISE STRATEGIES

"While taking care of a baby, running after a two-year-old, and dealing with life in general, I have one huge problem: When do I exercise and how do I find the energy for it when I have already used every ounce I have?" —K.S.

"Trade baby-sitting with a friend who will watch your children while you work out. Then you can baby-sit for your friend when she needs to do something."

"If you have no one who can watch your children, try going for a walk with them. They will probably have a blast, and you will be getting your workout and some quality time."

"*I* have a 13-month-old and I felt I had to wait until she went to bed at night to pull out my aerobics tapes. But I found that when I pop in the Tae Bo tape, her eyes are either glued to the screen or she's running around doing her own dance moves. The basic tape is only 30 minutes long and before you know it, it's time to cool down. You could probably squeeze this in when your baby takes a nap, even if it's a short one. Or if you have a younger baby, he can lie on the floor with his toys while you kick away."

"*A* gym with day care is a good investment. We end up
spending about $14 per week on the gym, and when you
figure how much the day care would cost, and all you
get from the gym, it is really worth the money."

"*S*o what if you can't spend 30 minutes on the treadmill?
Throw that laundry in the dryer! Beat those rugs! Get
it all out and then pat yourself on the back about how
much better you feel because you got a good workout
doing the housework."

Focus on healthy eating

*"Does anyone have any advice on how to start
losing the baby weight? I'm constantly hungry and
craving bad stuff."*—M.W.

"*J*ust go slow. I know I have my entire life to lose weight. If I lose too quickly, I may not maintain it. I have to start healthy habits, and each week I can get better and better. It's not an all-or-nothing race."

"*E*at only when you're hungry, and stop when you are full. Focus on activities instead of focusing on what you will eat for lunch. The more you shape your actions, the more you will become a part of those actions. And remember, there is nothing wrong with who you are right now. You are unique and special. It is your actions that need changing, not who you are."

"Start journaling what you eat. It might seem like a hassle, but if you do it for a couple of days, it will give you a good idea of what and how much you're eating. Then you can make any necessary adjustments."

"I crave junk food, mainly sweets and chocolate. Whenever I get a yearning for something unhealthy, I make myself drink water, as much as I can, and then go outside with the children. My baby loves it outside, and this helps to distract me from my cravings."

"If you are hungry, you should eat. It is your body telling you it needs more, and you need to listen. But instead of reaching for the chips or ice cream (my personal favorite), grab an apple. If you are nursing, you are feeding a whole other person right now, who is growing at an unbelievable rate, and you need to feed yourself and your baby. Just feed yourself the right thing and you'll stop being so hungry and will start to lose weight."

CHAPTER 3

How to Manage the New Family Dynamics

❧

"The year after our baby was born was so hard on my husband and me. We went through blame games and power struggles and all kinds of fun stuff. And then when we finally decided to work together on it, it was like a light went on and we both felt hope. And I stopped feeling like I was broken. Because we weren't broken, we were changing. And change, as scary as it may be, doesn't have to be bad."

EXPECT YOUR RELATIONSHIP TO CHANGE

"Things have changed so much between my husband and me since the baby came. How do I make us work as a couple, now that there are three of us?" —K.H.

"Your relationship with your husband will not be the same as it was before you had kids, but it will evolve into something wonderful. I sometimes still miss how it was with my husband before our first child was born. But if it weren't for us finding each other, our kids wouldn't exist. Now that's a deep thought."

"I find that I don't always treat my husband as if he were my best friend, which he is. So now I try to think of how I would respond to him if he were one of my girlfriends."

"The first year after having a baby is just plain hard—you're not getting any sleep, you don't know what to do with the baby, your body is whacked out. Your relationship with your husband is bound to change; whether it's for better or worse depends on the day. Just know that you're normal. Countless other couples have gone through that first year and come out even better: stronger, more confident, and more in love. That knowledge can help you make it through this time."

" *I* find that I have to remind myself that I am not my husband's mother. I am his wife, best friend, confidante, lover, and life partner."

" *I* am finally learning that being appreciative for what my husband does and asking for his help works much better than nagging. For example, I compliment him on how nice the yard looks after he's been raking, or I'll ask him nicely to empty the dishwasher. I've found that the more we show appreciation for each other, the less we argue."

GIVE YOUR HUSBAND BONDING TIME WITH THE BABY

"What can I do to help my husband feel involved now that we've got a new baby? I know there is so much to handle and sometimes I worry about him." —A.L.

"Guys like to be in charge of things. But when a new baby comes home, there's absolutely nothing they can control. Give your husband specific responsibilities: Sending the birth announcements. Making phone calls. Taking the official pictures of your baby's first months. Painting the baby's room. And then let him be in charge. Don't second-guess his decisions, just trust that he will make the right ones and relax."

"My husband grew distant after our first was born. He had a lot of fears he wasn't telling me about. When he finally opened up and talked about it he felt a lot better. Men are hard to figure out sometimes, and trying to get them to talk is like pulling teeth. So it may be up to you to keep asking questions so he'll talk about what's going on."

"When my son was a baby, he would start screaming every time my husband came near me. I had my husband spend more bonding time with the baby. It even helped with our love life: When we wanted some romantic time, I made sure the baby had everything he needed to be comfortable. I would let him relax in his swing for a while, sing him a song and put him down to sleep, turn on the monitor, and go back to my husband. As soon as the baby fell asleep, it was our turn."

"My husband works long hours and goes to graduate school two nights a week. But every night, we put the baby to sleep in our bed. We lie down together, and my husband reads *Goodnight Moon* while I nurse the baby to sleep. It's good for all of us, but especially my husband because it helps him feel connected to us even when he's on the go."

"To help my husband bond with our baby, I encouraged him to take over bath time so that he has a ritual that is all his own. He also sets aside at least an hour a night to have time alone with our baby—and I get the hour off!"

GET YOUR HUSBAND TO SHARE THE LOAD

"I have been looking forward to going back to work one day a week. I was shocked when my husband asked me not to. After we talked for a bit, he confided that he was afraid to be left alone with the baby. How can I get him to be my partner in parenting?" —E.G.

"My husband was afraid of taking care of the baby at first. So I started slowly: I left the baby with him while I went to do some errands for 30 minutes, then for an hour, then a couple of hours. After a little while, he found his own ways of soothing our son. Sometimes he's better at it than I am now."

"Sometimes, all you need to get help is to ask for it. Be very clear and loving in your requests, and your husband just might surprise you. As my grandmother used to say, 'Don't ask, don't get.'"

"My husband and I worked out a schedule: On
weeknights I take care of the baby myself. On Friday
and Saturday nights, he does it all. Defining who's
supposed to be doing what and when has helped with a
lot of the glaring and slamming doors I used to do when
I felt he wasn't doing his share."

"Including your husband in little decisions and
encouraging him to be part of the whole process will
go a long way toward making him feel he is an equal
partner. Ask for his opinions and take some of
his advice."

"My husband and I have a deal regarding dinner. Whoever gets home first will start dinner, and the other parent can play with the baby. After dinner the non-cooking parent gets to clean up while the other parent gets time with the kids before bed. It really does relieve some stress, and neither one of us feels like we are doing all the work."

DEAL WITH INTRUSIVE FAMILY MEMBERS

"What do you do about crazy in-laws? I know it's exciting to be grandparents, but ever since our son was born they have constantly made excuses to come over and tell me what to do." —R.M.

"*P*ut your mother-in-law to work. My mother-in-law watches the baby once a week so my husband and I can go on dates. At first, I was a little worried to leave our baby, but now I am so thankful."

"*G*et your husband to referee. He can take the weight of hospitality off you, and then you don't have to feel guilty if you need to excuse yourself to go lie down. Most in-laws aren't seeking to cause you hardship—they just have no clue where their boundaries are. Have your husband explain how they can help in a way that is truly helpful, not torturous."

"*My* mother-in-law gets on my nerves, but I force myself to remember that she means well and she loves me, my children, and my husband more than anything. I owe her respect for each of those things. Remember that your relationship with her has undergone a drastic change. You are no longer just her son's wife—you're the mother of her grandchildren. No matter what happens in your married life, you will always have a tie to this woman."

"My mother-in-law usually calls before coming over, so I just don't answer the phone. Also, I don't answer the door unless I'm expecting someone. I know that might sound rude, but sometimes I just want to be left alone."

"Practice this phrase: 'Thank you for your concern.' Honestly, it just does no good to engage an intrusive family member. I could try to justify my actions to my mother-in-law until I'm blue in the face, and she wouldn't change her mind. I just gave up after a while, and now I thank her for her concern and carry on as I was."

CHAPTER 4

How to Make Loving Fun Again

"We had to completely re-map my erogenous zones after the baby was born. What used to send me through the roof now just turns me off. And things that wouldn't have even mildly aroused me before are now a complete and total turn-on. Don't discount the idea that perhaps your switches have been rewired."

RECLAIM YOUR SEXUAL SELF

*"I'm married to an incredible man. He's very
supportive, helpful, romantic, and, well . . . horny.
I just don't feel like a sexual woman. Instead I feel
like an overweight housewife and mother. Any
suggestions?" —M.A.*

"*I* was really determined to get over feeling droopy and riddled with stretch marks. So I'm into lingerie now. I never bothered with it before, but now it definitely makes me feel sexy. "

"*F*or me the best aphrodisiacs are feeling well rested and knowing that my man is helping me. My husband now realizes that when he feels things are lacking in the intimacy department he can take on some obvious household chore like washing the dishes or cleaning the bathroom, or whisk the kids away on a weekend morning so I can sleep in peace for an extra hour or two. It works wonders for my libido. "

"After almost two years of trying everything, from doctors to antidepressants, I finally found the answer to my lack of libido. I started to go to the gym three days a week. It was amazing. Less than a week later, I started feeling like my old self again. I am by no means in great shape, but I don't feel like that overworked, overweight, housewife-mother woman I did before. Our sex life is getting back on track and it feels nice."

"Sexiness comes from within. Look in your heart and see yourself—a life-giver, a wife, a working woman, a human being. Wow, how beautiful."

"When you become a mom, your whole self-image changes. We have this image of our mothers, grandmothers, and all the purity and goodness that goes with motherhood. And suddenly being among those ranks, sex becomes less of a priority for us—we're moms now. Before we had children, who thought moms 'got nasty'? We have to redefine our thinking. Because if mothers were saints, they wouldn't be mothers."

$\mathcal{G}$ET PAST YOUR FEARS OF THE "FIRST TIME"

"I'm still a little traumatized by how different my body feels, especially 'down there.' How many attempts will it take before sex is comfortable and enjoyable again? Is there any way to avoid the pain?" —M.W.

"Don't expect perfection the first time (or the second or the third). You have to ease back into a sex life. Most important, don't worry. The more you worry, the worse it will be. Just take it one night at a time."

"Our son is seven months old, and it still isn't comfortable for me to have sex, at least without a lubricant. I was extremely skeptical about using a lubricant. But my husband really thought I should try it, and he was right. It is very natural-feeling, and it works wonders."

"My husband really helped ease me back into a healthy sex life. When we had sex for the first time, it was very painful and I was hesitant to try again. He was very gentle and didn't think about pleasuring himself for a few weeks. Instead, he just brought me to orgasm without intercourse and let me remember how to enjoy myself."

"When sex is painful, don't force yourself. Do it when you're ready physically and mentally. Then, both you and your husband will enjoy the lovemaking. It's worth the waiting. Meanwhile, remain intimate with plenty of hugs and kisses."

"Try letting yourself go. Say, 'The heck with it, I'm just going to do it.' I had to psych myself up a bit at first, and it helped. Talking honestly with my husband was also helpful. Most men are natural problem solvers. They want to help, plus they need the intimacy as much as we do."

REKINDLE THE ROMANCE

"My husband and I haven't spent a single night together alone since the baby was born. We are definitely feeling the effect of this on our marriage. How can we feel close again?" —M.M.

"Go soak in the tub and visualize everything you want in the picture of your intimate relationship. Make it the most loving, romantic, giving, fulfilling, vibrant marriage and relationship you can imagine. Start there and then you can work on making that new image happen."

"Make dates to do little things for each other, such as: 'Tomorrow morning, I'll give you a quick back massage.' Or, 'Let me prepare a bath for you tomorrow night.' You need each other's assurance right now that you will continue to make an effort during this rough time."

"My husband and I get a bottle of wine and some fancy, sinful treats from the bakery. We light some candles, put on some music that doesn't involve big purple dancing dinosaurs, and simply enjoy each other's company."

"We rent or buy books on tape or tapes of old scary radio shows. We turn off the lights, light some candles, and snuggle on the couch with some wine and listen. It's fun and more romantic to turn off the TV and let your ears and your imagination do some work for a change."

"My husband and I began a tradition of having an in-house date every Saturday night when our daughter was three months old. It was hard at first—we were both exhausted and just wanted to go to sleep. However, we both ended up enjoying ourselves. We light candles, dress up, and eat together—no matter how late it is after the kids have gone to sleep. We talk, hold hands, and exchange kisses during dinner. Then we cuddle on the couch and talk. Sometimes it leads to more; other times it doesn't."

COMMUNICATE YOUR NEW NEEDS AND DESIRES

"I can't be alone in this! I feel so self-conscious about sex. My husband thinks it's his fault, so it just keeps going in a vicious circle." —M.P.

"Be open with your husband about it, because he probably has no clue that your body has changed. All he knows is that he used to touch you one way and now it doesn't have the same effect, and he'll think it's him. Or that there's something wrong with you. In fact, it's neither."

"I need a little time to myself to help transition from 'mom' to 'hot mama.' Taking care of my baby all week drains me and doesn't put me in the mood to respond to my husband's legitimate needs for my undivided attention. I've noticed that my frame of mind improves and I am not as crabby if I just have a little time all alone."

"Check out John Gray's book *Mars and Venus in the Bedroom*. My husband and I started reading it after the birth of our second child. It helped immensely. We read it together and tried not to get offended by what the other person said. We found out a lot about each other, as well as opened some lines of communication about sex. We can now talk openly about it without getting our feelings hurt."

"Go for the cuddle factor in foreplay. Sometimes rather than wanting the hot and heavy foreplay, especially when we aren't feeling too sexy, being held and loved and cherished can be a big turn-on."

"My husband and I have both made compromises. For example, he's working at not throwing sexual hints at me all the time. I've told him that for me to get in the mood, I have to be able to be close to him without being afraid he's going to ask me for sex. He's also really working on being more loving outside the bedroom. It's easier when I feel like he wants to be with me, not just have sex."

CHAPTER 5

How to Cope When the Going Gets Tough

~

"As women, we put a lot of stress on ourselves, and this transfers to our kids. When you want to cry because it all seems so hard, wipe your tears and hold your precious baby. She loves you unconditionally—that is enough to get your heart going again in the right direction. Babies are amazing spirit lifters."

KNOW THAT THERE ARE GOOD DAYS AND BAD DAYS

"Is it just me or are others struggling to keep up with all that is expected of us? I just can't seem to get the hang of taking care of my son, picking up after my husband, working full-time outside the house, cooking and cleaning and doing laundry. My mom says it will get easier, but I need to know when!" —S.G.

"There are good days and bad, and I hit spots where I feel like I just can't do this anymore. When I get like that I try to do something special with my daughter, like picking up sandwiches and eating in the park. When I see how excited she gets, it puts everything in perspective. The laundry and housework will always be there, but she will only be little once."

"This is the time that you need friends the most. You don't need to struggle with your feelings of being overwhelmed alone. Call your friends, tell them how you're feeling, and ask for their advice and support."

"Write down everything that needs to get done and estimate how long it takes to do each thing. Then take the list and split it up with your husband or partner. I swear, until you do this, your husband has no idea how much you are doing to keep the household running."

"If you have the money, hire someone to clean your house. You work hard even if you never leave the house, and you deserve it. Just think of the time it will free up for other, more enjoyable activities."

"Try to take things just one hour at a time, even minute by minute if you have to. Focus on the good parts of your new life. Find whatever solace you can in your new routines and try to enjoy that part of it."

STOP PUTTING YOURSELF UNDER SO MUCH STRESS

"Anyone else feel like they aren't giving their babies enough attention? My husband is traveling, and between getting the stuff done around the house and just trying to get 15 minutes to myself during the day to get a shower and something to eat, I feel like I am never doing enough for my kids." —E.M.

"This may sound crazy, but talk with your little one and tell her that you will try your best to be the best mommy and that you love her and that you both will grow together. It really took pressure off me when I told my daughter that I wanted to do what was best and not stress us both out. I know that sounds silly, but just talking to their calm little faces really helps."

"I spend so much time thinking about my kids and worrying about everything. As easy as it is to tell yourself, 'Don't worry,' I know how hard it is to actually do. I've made a conscious effort in my life to relax by taking yoga classes. This lets me spend two hours each week not thinking about anything but myself. It's wonderful."

"This mom thing never gets easy. You get used to it, but it's not ever easy. Relax. Just drop the worry and the guilt. I'm speaking from experience. If you let it eat you up, you won't be able to enjoy anything."

"All moms worry. It's in our nature. Try to relax and enjoy every minute you have with your baby. Somehow babies can tell when we're uptight, and it just gets them uptight as well. Take a deep breath and take it one day at a time. Everything always has a way of falling into place and working out beautifully, and when it doesn't go perfectly, it's a great opportunity to learn."

"Try to use your common sense. I know it's hard when your hormones are raging. Once my son started sleeping through the night, he'd wake up in the morning and wouldn't eat much at all. I thought something was wrong until I finally figured out that he just doesn't like to eat as soon as he awakes. He needs some time in the morning to wake up, just like his daddy does. What I thought was a crisis was just an opportunity to learn more about my baby's personality and adjust accordingly."

DEAL WITH BREASTFEEDING SETBACKS

"Every time I think breastfeeding is going well, something seems to go wrong: The baby won't nurse or even latch on, or the pain starts again. I'm stressed and my breasts hurt and I'm crying all the time. I can't bear to think about giving up nursing. I know it's silly, considering it's upsetting me so much, but my heart just breaks when I think of giving it up. Any advice?" —E.S.

"*I*f you're having trouble breastfeeding, contact a lactation consultant (if you haven't already). They can truly make all the difference. They can point out one or two things that make breastfeeding a much more enjoyable experience."

"*B*reastfeeding didn't work out for us. I felt so guilty that I cried every time I made a bottle or saw a mother breastfeeding. It was awful. Then I started to notice how much happier my baby was after I weaned her. She didn't have thrush, latching problems, or as much reflux. She was gaining weight nicely and was a calmer baby. My poor nipples finally healed, I got more sleep, and I was happier, too. Now I look back and wonder why I stood it so long."

"*I* felt like such a failure when I had problems breastfeeding. I thought it was natural and didn't understand why I couldn't do it easily and comfortably. My lactation consultant pointed out that breastfeeding is a learned behavior, and reassured me that I couldn't be expected to know how to breastfeed without instruction and support. Most women need to seek out quality support and information to learn the basics of breastfeeding. I felt so much better when I realized I wasn't to blame."

"Although breastfeeding is great for a baby's health, so is having a mother who is sane and feels good. You can't help your baby if you are crying and depressed all the time."

"It isn't your fault that breastfeeding isn't going well. With my first baby I had many breastfeeding problems. I eventually stopped breastfeeding and then felt horrible about it. With my second baby, it was a totally different story—I had a supportive environment and knowledgeable health-care professionals to help me. Don't beat yourself up if you decide to stop breastfeeding. It's understandable if you are in pain. But you might not need to if you get the right help."

$\mathcal{A}$SK FOR HELP WHEN YOU NEED IT

"I am going crazy. I am weepy and grouchy all the time. I just feel so overwhelmed and exhausted that I don't know what to do. Is it normal to feel this way postpartum, or is it something more?" —S.E.

"Does your family know how you are feeling? Is there someone you can confide in that you trust to give you an honest, objective opinion about how you're feeling? I think that if you are feeling bad enough to wonder if you're depressed, you know that something isn't quite right. Listen to your heart. It doesn't hurt to tell others what you're feeling. In fact, you will feel so much better afterward. Call on your network of support."

"I waited a long time before I got help because I kept thinking I wasn't depressed. I thought being depressed meant feeling sad and crying all the time. But that's not how everyone reacts to it. If you feel really out of sorts, go get some help even if you aren't 'sad.'"

"*I* don't think it matters if what you have is the baby blues, postpartum depression, or just plain old depression. If your depression is severe, call your doctor. If you can still function, you'll feel better if you go out and do something. Call a friend and have lunch together, or see if there is anyone who can come over and watch your kids for two hours while you take a nap or do something just for yourself."

"*P*ostpartum depression can strike at any time. One of the first things you should do is get a medical evaluation to determine if there is a physical cause for the problem. Go have a complete physical. And do it with a doctor you trust. Be honest about your symptoms. I say that because I wasn't totally honest with my doctor and it delayed effective treatment for me."

"*D*on't wait to get help. Call your doctor. There is help out there to make you feel better. It took talking to a therapist to realize that although I loved my daughter and took great care of her, I felt like I was not connecting because I felt resentful for losing my past life. My therapist also helped me see that what I was feeling was a totally normal thing to go through. I can tell you, now that I have sought help I feel like my old self again. I have established a good routine with my family and feel settled."

CHAPTER 6

How to Handle Going Back to Work (or Not)

"*I* went back to work today for the first time in four months. It was hard. I talked to all my colleagues about how sad I had been to leave my baby this morning. I called home every hour. All in all, I didn't get much work done, but the day passed and tomorrow will be a little easier. And my son, of course, was absolutely fine when I got home."

$\mathcal{F}$IND THE RIGHT CHILD-CARE SITUATION

"How did you find child care? It seems like such a daunting task, and I would love some guidance." —A.S.

"First, interview a minimum of three child-care centers and see how they compare to one another. Second, find out if they are licensed by the state, which will give you assurance that they meet minimum standards. Next, cover the following with each center: How do the caregivers discipline the children? (Although this is not pertinent to babies, it will become more important as your child grows.) What kind of routine is set up? How often are children fed and changed? Finally, go to observe the center. Watch the interactions between the caregivers and the babies. Do they seem loving and attentive? Is the space clean? Are the toys clean and in good condition? What is the visitation policy? Is visiting encouraged or discouraged?"

"*E*xtensive interviews with other parents who use a specific caretaker were the most helpful when we were making our selection. Make a list of questions and bring it with you when you visit the center. I also dropped by unannounced a few times. It was the best indicator of how things were going."

"*W*hen you are in the center, use your senses. Do you see happy children, or do you hear lots of crying? Do the caregivers seem to enjoy their work, or do they look stressed out? Put yourself in your child's little shoes. They will be spending the bulk of their day there. Is it a place you would feel happy to be for eight or more hours every day? If you feel good about the child-care center, it's likely your child will feel good about it, too. Just take your time, do your homework, and trust your intuition."

"I called the Better Business Bureau and the state child-care licensing department. They told me how many complaints had been filed for a specific child-care center, what the complaint was regarding, and what the resolution was. It was a great source of information."

"When I interviewed child-care providers, I asked for names of references and spoke with parents of other children who were in their care. It was helpful to me to talk to people whose children had been cared for by them. For instance, one provider I was checking out had clients who liked her but expressed some reservations about her style—too structured, and so on. The question 'Would you choose this child-care provider to watch your children if you were doing it over?' elicited good, honest responses."

FACE YOUR OWN SEPARATION ANXIETY

"I am sad about leaving my baby. Are there any hints on how to get prepared for going back to work?" —M.F.

"Begin dropping your baby at child care several weeks before you go back to work. My daughter went to child care the same day I returned to work, and it was awful. My daughter adjusted fine, but I was a mess. I couldn't think and was so upset because it was the first time we'd been apart since she was born. Keep her there for half-days for the first week. When you go to pick her up you may want to stay another hour just so you can watch the teachers interact with the children. That will help both of you adjust. Then, begin full days the second week."

"*If* you are close enough, visit your child-care center during your lunch hour. Those occasional lunchtime visits make a world of difference for me. I also have brought the baby to my work space. I have a set of plastic frames to rotate the most current baby pictures. It entertains my coworkers, too. If your workplace is amenable, scan some photos and use them as the wallpaper on your computer."

"*Try* to ease back into the working world by starting part-time. I did a 50 percent work schedule for a month and then 75 percent for eight weeks before going back to full-time. Those extra couple of hours made a big difference while adjusting to being back at work."

"*I* found talking to other women at work who have young children tremendously helpful. I've actually become quite close to a couple of ladies at work, and they're such wonderful moms that they inspire me. It helps to see that their kids are doing great and that it can be done."

"*F*or those first few days or weeks back, don't expect anything of yourself other than going to work, going home, and having baby time. Either make and freeze enough meals to sustain yourself, or hit the frozen food section of your supermarket. Buy a pack of paper plates and don't think about the dishes until you've used them up."

*F*IGURE OUT IF PUMPING IS FOR YOU

*"I am returning to work in one week and am
nervous about keeping up with breastfeeding.
When do you pump? How will I have enough of
a supply to keep my baby full and happy? Any
advice?"* —D.T.

"Try not to worry. It won't solve anything and will only make you tense, which your baby can sense. You either will have enough milk to feed your baby and your worries will have been in vain, or you won't have enough milk and your baby will have to learn to enjoy formula—and there's nothing you could have done about it anyway. As long as you do everything with love, your baby will thrive as he should."

"Pump every chance you get. Pump even if your baby has just eaten and nothing comes out. It will help to build up your milk supply. At first, it was painful as either the baby or the pump was on my breasts all the time. But it worked. Just pump, pump, pump. Then when you get tired, pump some more."

"*I* was forced to supplement and it's really not that bad. The important thing is that your baby gets enough to eat and hopefully some of it is breast milk. Pumping is not natural and it takes a bit of getting used to. Try looking at your baby or a picture of your baby. Visualize your baby breastfeeding while you are pumping. Don't think about the pump or how much milk you're getting; instead, read a magazine, surf the Web, or catch up on phone calls."

"Arrange for a comfortable, private place at work for pumping. Be sure to pump at the same time every day at work, preferably coinciding with your baby's feeding pattern so your supply and your baby's needs are in sync on weekends. If you need to, reserve your normal pumping times in your calendar as regular appointments."

"If you're cool and matter-of-fact about pumping, or better yet, have a sense of humor about it, you might be surprised at how well your coworkers will accommodate you. I even ended up making some business contacts while pumping alongside another mom in the ladies' room at a trade show."

*P*UT COWORKERS' COMPLAINTS TO REST

*"I can see my coworkers' eyes roll when I have to
leave a meeting early to be sure to get to the
child-care center to pick up my son. What's the
best way to deal with their resentment?"* —S.R.

"*I* work two days a week. Frankly, some of my coworkers are resentful, and they sometimes make cracks about my schedule. My usual response is to laugh it off. I also recognize that some people are jealous and wish they could do what I'm doing. So I try to work extra hard and be willing to take on less-than-desirable projects so that I make myself valuable."

"*O*ur receptionist kept commenting on what time I left at night. Things like, 'Oh, you're leaving early again.' So I addressed it with her. I said, 'It really bothers me when you make comments regarding what time I leave at night. Please don't do it anymore.' She was stunned. Later, she came to my office and apologized and thanked me for telling her how I felt."

"You may need to sit down and discuss whatever issues your coworkers might have with your family obligations. And it might be as enlightening for you as it is for them. They may not be quite as critical as you think they are—I know when I am tired and stressed, I oftentimes blow stuff out of proportion."

"If someone is really giving you a hard time, have lunch with her one day. You could explain your situation and talk about what a huge difference having the flexibility to leave to pick up your child has made in your life. Then address ways that you both can have your work needs met."

"My advice is to take a soft yet direct approach. Tell any critics how important it is for you to be able to keep your schedule and then ask them to address any of their concerns directly with you. It is hard for someone to ignore a direct request, and sugarcoating it just won't help in these situations. When it comes to protecting your schedule, you need to be direct."

$\mathcal{N}$EGOTIATE FOR MORE FLEXIBILITY

"I would really like to work a shorter week when I return from maternity leave. Does anyone have any creative ways of spending less time at the office while still completing all the responsibilities of your job?" —R.K.

"Check out the Website www.workoptions.com. It outlines flexible work schedules and how to ask your boss for one. I used one of their kits to create a proposal to work a 30-hour week, and it worked."

"I wrote a flextime proposal recently. I started off with, 'I would like to propose a change in my present work schedule that will allow me to maintain the commitment I've shown to the company over the past five years while giving me some needed flexibility.' The proposal included sections titled 'Why I'm Confident This Will Work for the Company' and 'Contingency Plans.' I outlined my responsibilities and hours in the office under 'Specifics.' It worked!"

"*P*resent your boss with a compelling argument for why your working at home would benefit the company, and why you would continue to perform your job as well as, if not better than, before. Think of the issues she'll bring up and address them as part of this talk. Set up a trial period, and agree on a date when you two will get together to evaluate how the trial went. Let her know that you'll respect whatever decision she makes and that your performance will not be affected if she disagrees with you. You might just be surprised at the outcome."

"*I* recently requested a laptop computer so that I can work when I'm at home. If the laptop idea won't fly, ask your company to provide you with any software you may need to install on your home PC so that you can easily work from home when you are there."

"*Many* employers don't believe that you will actually be working from home if you don't have someone at home with you to care for the baby. If you are thinking of proposing a schedule that includes working from home, make sure you have help lined up, and then be sure to tell your employer that you would have someone with you to care for the baby, leaving you free to focus on your work."

$\mathscr{A}$LLOW YOURSELF TO CONSIDER STAYING AT HOME

"I am having second thoughts about going back to work. I dread the idea of leaving my daughter. Is it crazy for me to think about staying home instead?" —R.R.

"If you really want to try staying at home but want to minimize the risk, ask your employer for an unpaid leave of absence for a few months. Then if it doesn't work out, you can always go back to work."

"Having been both a working mom and a stay-at-home mom, I have realized I have more to offer my kids when I am not working. The stress level in our home plummeted when I finally got to stay home. The kids don't know how much is in our savings, and they don't care if their clothes come from Wal-Mart or the mall. Best of all, I feel much closer to my children than before."

"*R*esearch what it will actually cost for you to work. How much will you spend on child care, car expenses, meals out, and work clothing? Many families find that not having to pay for child care, being in a different tax bracket, and implementing some cost-cutting strategies allow them to live on one income comfortably."

"*I*f you want to make staying at home economically feasible, start giving up the little things. My husband and I have been enjoying a comfortable lifestyle, and we indulge in a lot of extras. One of the first things I gave up was getting my nails done. I also take my lunch to work. At the end of the week I transfer what I would have spent on those things into savings. I hope that these little things will add up fast and we will develop a nice nest egg in savings. Then, hopefully, we'll see that we don't really need my salary."

"Staying at home with your child for a few years doesn't mean giving up your career forever. Use the time at home to reevaluate how your career aspirations fit with your new life. If you discover that you miss your job, you will find a way to go back. Or you might decide that you want a different career now that you are a mother. I realized that, although I enjoyed the financial rewards of my job, once my son goes to preschool I want to go back to work in a field that provides greater emotional satisfaction and that will accommodate my child's schedule."

$\mathcal{A}$DJUST TO LEAVING YOUR JOB

"I always thought I wanted to stay home when I had a baby, so I quit a job I absolutely loved. I had no idea that I would experience such an emotional change. I can say, without a shadow of a doubt, motherhood is the hardest job I've ever had. How can I ease the transition?" —C.W.

"*If* you really miss your career, keep a foot in the door. Take classes or seminars to keep yourself up-to-date. You are entitled to change your mind if going back to work would make you happier. A happy mom leads to a happy family. Be open to the possibility that you might go back sooner than you had ever thought."

"*Try* to approach being a stay-at-home mom as a job and set personal goals to keep you motivated. You have this precious time when you don't have to spend 40 hours a week at work. What would you like to accomplish? When you were working, what did you dream of being able to do at home? Even if it is cleaning out that closet, starting a new exercise regimen, or learning how to make homemade bread, now is the time to indulge in those dreams."

"*O*ne of the reasons I was picking fights with my husband, rolling my eyes at him, and sometimes being downright nasty to him was that I was resentful of his having a career while I had to stay home all day. Now, he encourages me to get out of the house and to take time for myself. Slowly things are getting better between us. And better with me."

"*Y*ou could get your feet wet with a part-time position. It gives you the chance to prove yourself and gain confidence in the new situation, as well as transition your baby gradually into a child-care situation. Once you feel confident in your job skills and balancing ability, you can make a decision about what to do from there."

"There are long stretches of time when I feel like I've given up every personal goal and sacrificed myself for my family, and I resent it. And there are days when I call my husband and tell him, 'I quit!' But then there are days when I roll around on the bed with my daughter all morning. I am the one she wants and needs when she is hurt, sick, or scared. I know what she's watching, who she's playing with. I am her safe place. And when she grows up, she will always know that I was here for her."

CHAPTER 7

How to Still Have a Life

~

"*L*ive your life normally and go where you need to go. Now you just have a diaper bag and baby to take along. This helps children learn early how to behave in public. In addition, letting children know they are not being left behind helps them develop a sense of belonging and safety."

SEEK OUT ADULT INTERACTION

"I have spent the first 10 months of my son's life at home with him, and I honestly feel as if my mind is oozing out of my ears. I am crying for some stimulating adult conversation. How can I find it?" —M.O.

"Visit friends, neighbors, or relatives at their homes,
or invite them over to yours. Just make a light lunch or
dessert and invite them over for conversation."

"Set up play dates so your baby will be engaged but you
can interact with other moms. If you haven't found
another mom yet, put a sign up in your neighborhood
and see what happens!"

"*T*ake a night class, even if it isn't academic. Something like yoga, swimming, art, sewing, or cooking."

⌒⌒

"*V*olunteer at a hospital, the Red Cross, or a school. If you are really in need of an outlet, this will not cost you anything and will give you a nice feeling of contributing to society."

"*I* don't know what I would do without the Internet and message boards. My family lives six hours away and I have no friends in town—yet. But thanks to the message boards, I had someone to whine to when my back hurt, when I was lonely, when I was afraid of labor. And after the children were born, I had friends to share milestones with, and to turn to for information, support, and advice. I think the message boards are the fences of our modern day where women can gossip, share recipes, commiserate, and have adult interaction."

*F*IND A GOOD SITTER

*"How did you find someone you felt comfortable
with to baby-sit your children?"* —K.M.

"It's all about using your community. Get to know your neighbors with kids. Find out if there are any au pairs in your neighborhood, because they usually don't work past 7:00 P.M."

"When you find someone you like, sit down and ask her: 'How would you deal with an emergency? What would you do if my child woke up crying? How would you handle discipline?' If you're comfortable with her answers, the kids like her, and she's got good references, agree on a price and enjoy your night out."

"*If* you are unsure about a new baby-sitter, have her come and help you at the house one day. Then move to going out for a cup of coffee, or something that you won't be gone too long for. Before you know it, you will be more comfortable with her."

"*Call* the Red Cross and ask for referrals of young teens who have taken its baby-sitting course. They learn first aid, basic principles of child development, how to prepare simple snacks, and fun games."

"Try finding someone who is interested in swapping baby-sitting hours. Every other Tuesday I watch a friend's son for three hours, and she watches my daughter on the alternate Tuesdays. It's a great way for me to get time to run errands or nap, something I can always use. And my baby is getting some playtime."

STAY IN TOUCH WITH FRIENDS

"How do you find the time to devote to friendships? I can't seem to make this work. By the time I do everything I need to do, I never have the time or energy to pursue other relationships." —M.T.

"*I* found that I needed to get my husband's attention and enlist his help. Now I tell him, 'I really need your help in making time for me to meet with my friends.' We agree to a time where he will take care of our son while I go out."

"*If* your friends don't have babies, don't babble on about your child unless your friend asks. A once-a-week-or-so update is good. Any more than that can bore them, and they will get tired of hearing about it."

"Sometimes I would feel too tired to even call my friends on the phone. I'd always think, I'll do it tomorrow. I decided to set myself a phoning timetable. I'd make a phone call every other day and two on Sunday. I did that for a month, and I began to feel caught up. Also, phones do have two ends—when you call, people invariably say, 'I'm so sorry I haven't called.' So you're not the only person feeling neglectful."

"I think that to a certain degree if you want family time and work time, then friendships do suffer. There's only so much time to go around. So I have decided to devote time to three women I really like, and not feel guilty about the rest. Having time to spend quietly at home with my family compensates nicely."

"Take your little one along when you get together with friends. I had many a dinner with friends when my daughter was little. She would generally sleep through the meal, or would be happy to lie in my arms or be rocked in her carrier."

REMEMBER THAT YOU ARE STILL YOU

"I get so depressed sometimes because I feel like I am just a wife and a mom and nothing else. I feel like I lost a little bit of myself along the way. Anyone else feel like this?" —P.M.

"When you take the time to do things that you enjoy and have some alone time, you will be a happier person and a better mom. Think about the image we give our children when we don't take care of ourselves. How can our children respect us as people, and not just moms, if we don't let them see us respecting ourselves?"

"This is a little thing, but it goes a long way: Remember to introduce yourself by your name, not as 'so-and-so's mom.' I meet so many women at mothers' groups who never use their own names! Avoiding that habit has helped me remember I'm still a person in my own right."

"*W*henever I feel sorry for myself, I pick up an Anne Tyler novel. Almost any one will do. Because she's almost always celebrating family life and reminding you to take a step back when you think you've thrown your life away. You might find that you've got a pretty good life after all."

"*F*irst, know that you are not alone. Tons of other moms are feeling the exact same way. Second, be sure to talk to other adults about something other than feeding and pooping. Once you see that you do still have thoughts in your head beyond 'It's 45 minutes until the next feeding,' you will feel more like yourself."

"When I first became a mom, I was all about changing diapers and doing laundry every waking hour. Because I worked full-time, I felt guilty if I didn't dedicate 110 percent of my home time to my family. Finally, I realized that I couldn't give 110 percent to anyone because I wasn't giving anything to myself. That's when I set aside two hours each week for 'me time.' Sometimes I soak in the tub with a good book. Other times I just sleep in on a Saturday morning. Whatever I do, it helps me realize that life will go on a lot more smoothly if I take a couple of hours off from being a mom."

ABOUT NANCY EVANS

Nancy Evans is cofounder and editor in chief of iVillage, and a mother.

ABOUT iVILLAGE

Based in New York City, iVillage Inc. was founded in 1995 with the intention of "humanizing cyberspace." In the early years of the Internet, there were few places for women to find solutions and discuss their problems, needs, and interests. By providing a clean, well-lit space, iVillage carved out a unique place where women could gather and find information and support on a wide range of topics relevant to their lives.

Today, iVillage is a leading women's media company and the number one source for women's information online, providing practical solutions and everyday support for women. iVillage includes iVillage.com, Women.com, Business Women's Network, Lamaze Publishing, the Newborn Channel, iVillage UK, Promotions.com, and Astrology.com.

iVillage.com's content areas include Astrology, Babies, Beauty, Diet & Fitness, Entertainment, Food, Health, Home & Garden, Lamaze, Money, Parenting, Pets, Pregnancy, Relationships, Shopping, and Work.